Dissociative Effect

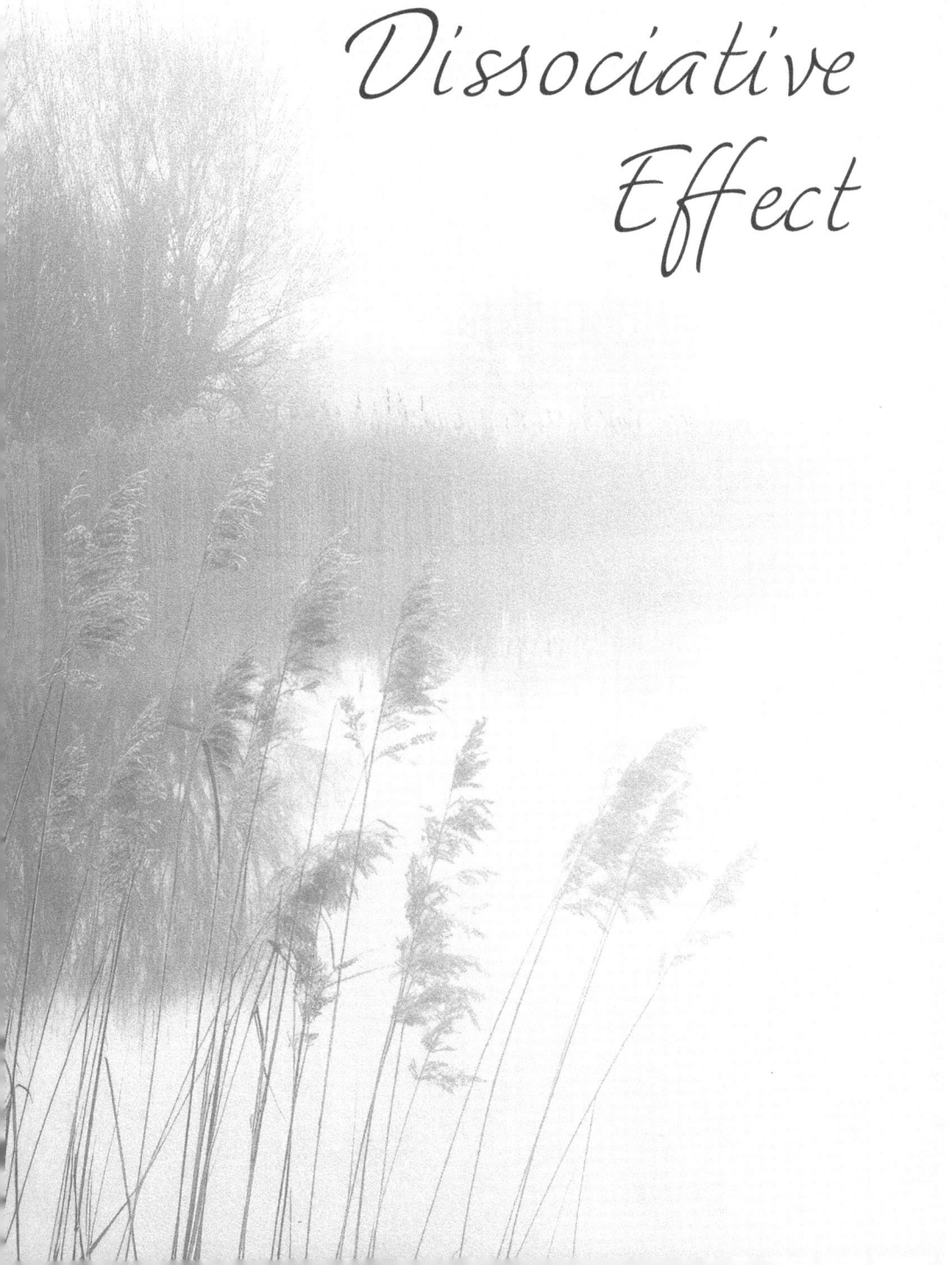

Dissociative Effect

poems by
Jacqueline S. Redmer, M.D.

SHANTI ARTS PUBLISHING
BRUNSWICK, MAINE

Dissociative Effect

Published by Shanti Arts LLC
193 Hillside Road
Brunswick, Maine 04011
shantiarts.com

Designed by Shanti Arts Designs

Cover image—Mini_AI / 838481284 / stock.adobe.com

Printed in the United States of America

ISBN: 978-1-962082-82-2 (softcover)

Library of Congress Control Number: 2025945841

To my girls . . .
May the sound of crickets against the blanket of a dark,
silent night remind you that you are never alone.

Contents

ad sanadum

Acknowledgments

I want to thank my husband, Thomas, for helping me to build a writing shed in the backyard. I also want to thank the cohort of therapists, friends, mentors, and spiritual teachers who graciously read the poems I sent out via email, understanding that a poem, like the heart of a person, needs to be seen or heard by at least one other person.

Introduction

I never wrote a poem until I was in my early forties. If you had asked me to do so, I would have said, "I'm a left-brained person." This was the story I told myself throughout my adult life until I found myself in a particular point of professional and personal unhappiness. In an effort to survive, I turned to writing— poetry in particular. I didn't know it at the time but I was in need of some new stories.

After seeing patients at work one day, I was in a mood of strong and overwhelming emotion. Somehow I had the spontaneous idea that I should write a poem—or rather that I needed to write a poem. This first poem was called "decomposition" and is included in this collection. In this poem a person describes the internal experience of slowly dying— decomposition—even as they outwardly appear to be living a normal life. The next day brought another poem and then unfolded two to three years of compulsive poetry writing. Over time I noticed that I would start writing a poem in a particular emotional state or mood, and by the end of writing the poem, I would feel something different.

It turns out that my experience with writing was not unique, and I was intuitively drawn to the healing benefits of expressive writing. Expressive writing is characterized as a form of intentional written emotional disclosure. Researchers have found that this form of writing doesn't only feel good, it also enhances people's physical and psychological health. There are over two thousand academic articles documenting the health effects of expressive writing, including benefits on immune function, sleep, mental health, and pain.

Neuroscientists have discovered that putting words to emotions calms the brain's fear response, strengthens emotional regulation, and even rewires neural pathways. Similar to trauma therapies like EMDR, expressive writing reduces activity in the amygdala (the fear center of the brain) and increases activity in the prefrontal cortex, the region of the brain responsible for logical thinking and self-regulation. In other words, writing gives the emotional brain a way to slow down and step back, which allows the thinking brain to take the lead. Instead of getting hijacked by feelings, writing lets you step outside of them, name them, and in doing so, change the way they affect you.

Inherent in the process of writing is also the organization and reorganization of cognitive and emotional content. This helps us to find meaning in our life experiences—a very important task for the human brain. Humans have evolved to depend on the collective and individual narratives that form the substrate of our lives. We think in stories, talk in stories, understand our future and past as stories while narrating an unfolding autobiography to our innerselves in stories. Humans are stories.

When we realize "we are made of stories," it stands to follow that we are the narrators, and we have the ability to change aspects of the stories that we have been telling ourselves. It was a healing process for me to learn that our lives are constructed narratives, a process I first encountered as a client in psychotherapy, then as an emerging poet, and then as a student and practitioner of narrative medicine. True to the saying, "energy flows where attention goes," we have the ability to shift the intention and quality of our lives.

According to social scientist James Pennebaker, Ph.D., there are aspects of intentional writing practice that are likely to make it more effective as a therapeutic intervention. Linguistic attempts to change perspective through pronoun shifting are associated with less depression and anxiety. The use of first-person singular pronouns, such as "I," can indicate a focus on oneself, and this is often linked to higher rates of anxiety, insecurity, or depression. "Perspective switching," reflected in pronoun shifts, is related to improved mental health. This involves reflecting on problems from different points of view by using "I," "you," "we," or "he/ she/they." With this advice in mind, we might consider the possibility that intentional writing has the potential to encourage changing perspectives and revising our stories, if we are willing to consider the different narrative voices of our lives.

On Dissociation

Dissociation often refers to a state of mind in which a person is disconnected from their bodies, thoughts, feelings, memories, or sense of reality. As humans this helps us to endure pain and trauma, which in the moment might otherwise seem unbearable. Although dissociation is often associated with clinical disorders, dissociative experiences are known to occur on a spectrum in the general population, perhaps owing   to differences in personality and neural processing. We can leave our bodies for a moment or for decades, and not even be aware of it.

"Dissociative effect" is the phrase often used in medicine when talking about a side effect of the drug ketamine. Ironically, the chemical properties of ketamine that induce dissociation can also increase neuroplasticity and provide therapeutic benefit for patients struggling with depression, post-traumatic stress disorder (PTSD), addiction, and other mental health issues. Although dissociative thought patterns can prevent people from fully inhabiting their lives, ketamine-assisted therapy has shown that psychedelics can also be a gateway past structured narratives and difficult-to-change cognitive patterns.

In this book of poetry, "dissociation" is a proxy for the distance one feels from living an embodied, authentic life. While this separation can be painful to appreciate, it also teaches us that our lives are constructed of narrative—the stories told by ourselves and to ourselves by others—and these narratives can change over time. The "dissociative effect" is also a reference to the perspective shifting that is a necessary part of healing and the wisdom that can come with aging. These movements within ourselves reveal vulnerabilities as well as doors to creativity, knowledge, and deeper longings.

In these poems, I explore my own experiences with disembodiment and my efforts to return to wholeness. I also reflect on stories I have heard in my work as a physician. I share these words, not to tell you about who I am, but, rather, as a deeper invitation into your own story. May these poems bring you back to places within yourself you have always known.

References

Lieberman, M. D. et al. "Putting Feelings into Words: Affect Labeling Disrupts Amygdala Activity in Response to Affective Stimuli." *Psychological Science* 18, no. 5 (2007): 421–428.
    Explains how writing about emotions reduces
    amygdala activity and strengthens emotional regulation.

Pennebaker, J. W. *Opening Up: The Healing Power of Expressing Emotions.* Guilford Press, 1997.
  A deep dive into expressive writing and how journaling can help with emotional processing, stress, and even physical health.

Pennebaker, J. W. and Beall, S. K. "Confronting a Traumatic Event: Toward an Understanding of Inhibition and Disease." *Journal of Abnormal Psychology* 95, no. 3 (1986): 274–281.
  A foundational study showing how writing about emotions leads to reduced stress and improved immune function.

Kross, E. et al. "Self-talk as a Regulatory Mechanism: How You Do It Matters." *Journal of Personality and Social Psychology* 106, no. 2 (2014): 304–324.
  Explores how journaling and self-reflection help regulate emotions by engaging the prefrontal cortex.

Emmons, R. A. and McCullough, M. E. "Counting Blessings Versus Burdens: An Experimental Investigation of Gratitude and Subjective Well-being in Daily Life." *Journal of Personality and Social Psychology* 84, no. 2 (2003): 377–389.
  Examines how gratitude journaling increases dopamine and serotonin, improving mood and well-being.

Smyth, J. M. et al. "Effects of Writing about Stressful Experiences on Symptom Reduction in Patients with Asthma or Rheumatoid Arthritis: A Randomized Trial." *Journal of the American Medical Association* 28, no. 14 (1999): 1304–1309.
  Shows how expressive writing leads to measurable physical health improvements.

Pathos

Entering the Belly of the Whale

—Necropsy, Scotland Outer Hebrides, November 28, 2019

The stench was overwhelming
as you entered into

bones, blubber, organs, gristle;
such a mess was left behind

when all peristalsis stopped—
you tried to rid yourself of

those indigestible plastic products
those islands of debris

covered in thick residues of shame;
while in the distance you heard laughter

and the explosion of cheap Chinese fireworks
littering the canvas of a perfect night sky.

the magician

the careful optics
of a sly smile
and you become
the illusion—the absence
of what one sees.

when you sit,
you are not the chair;
when you walk,
you are not the floor;
when the sun shines,
you might be the shadow,
but never the sun.

you know the empty space,
the loss of a memory,
the pause between words,
the softness of a sigh,
and even
the space between the fingertips
that hurt the softer parts of you—

or perhaps, such harm
never actually happened
because sometimes,
when you are in your body
you are not your body.

creation story

and then on the eighth day
God made a girl—
not a reflection of His image
but an object lesson
with man holding the authority
to consume her innocence
if desired, but not by her.
instead, he filled her basket
with the weight of guilt
taking the temptation she birthed
shaming any claim she made
to live in her own body.

on pleasure, this was true

the comfort of thumb sucking
        you remember—also the words
"take that thing out of your mouth,"
        taught you
about the necessity of secret pleasures
        and hiding, except sometimes
you couldn't hear them coming or
        you thought no one would notice
as your favorite appendage
        found its way
into your sleeping mouth
        even as they covered and painted
comfort with poison and hot pepper oil
        even as metal prongs were attached
to your palate by the dentist;
        such a strange cruelty imposed
when it was decided
        that the soft consolation
of your body be forgotten—
        they told you this was love
and such efforts would help you
        avoid a lifetime of orthodontia.

enough

"don't you think
you've had enough?"
they said,

food shaming your growing child's body
because you wanted more of—
something.

instead, on that day,
your cheeks burned and you filled up
with self-contempt instead.

your eyes survived by looking inward
believing the story
that you would never be enough.

you know now, if love isn't nurtured
then longing leaves a mark
on a girl too—

and empty becomes
enough.

on watching Mr. Roger's neighborhood, circa 1980

some people are able to imagine
places they have never been

just as farsickness whispers
with a distant pain

and memory invades with strange desire
of wanting to love and to be loved

and to be held
being held

in all the worlds of make believe
give us hope that this world is bearable

that it is ok to feel sad
for what was wanted but unavailable.

"The world is not always a kind place," he once said.
*"That's something all children learn for themselves,
  whether we want them to or not, but it's something they
  really need our help to understand."* —Fred Rogers

Prayers on Sunday

the DeAngelo family sits
in the front row of the Church.
my family, we were in the second row
every Sunday—

someone once told me
I was made in the image of God.
this, I contemplated and also how fat I felt
in those blue and green plaid pants

I was instructed to wear
feeding the growing distrust for my 12-year-old body.
I was told that girls should learn self-respect—
they should cover up with vertical stripes

so as to appear smaller.

I was told that sacrifice tests our faith
in God's ultimate wisdom;
then watched as my thoughts, my dreams
were bound, unseen and hiding

behind those vertical stripes.
I wanted to be saved
but I don't know if God saw me
with my head bowed and knees aching.

I couldn't see God at all
from the second row of the church.

Doe in the Snow

—inspired by "The Buck in The Snow"
by Edna St Vincent Millay

Doe in the snow. I found you
in the early winter twilight, resting
under a canopy of hoar frosted pine boughs
with your glass eyes and stiff body
frozen to the ground.

My fingers grazed your chest
feeling the wound which emptied you of life
your sinewy legs tangled
never again to frolic in fresh powder snow
or to prance through flowering summer fields.

My doe in the snow. Tell me—
was it shame or fear that made us run
when we had been hurt,
when we came to understand
this strange thing we found in ourselves
in this lonely life we created?

My doe in the snow. I saw you
as a hunter's indiscretion, aggression
just before he pulled the trigger
drinking his cheap beer and muttering
"those bitches are all the same."

My doe in the snow. You too must know
how strange a thing is pain. That day, I was wounded—
blood staining the whiteness of snow.
They say a girl should always heed winter warnings.
She should know better.

dis-comfort food

"put that back," they said,
        "that junk, will make you fat."

your throat swelled shame
and freckled cheeks burned crimson

maybe it was another day that brought the wisdom

        "nobody wants a fat girl."

you considered their words
putting those $0.25 Little Debbie Snack Cakes
back on the shelf of gas station comfort food

not understanding why some bodies were born good
and some bodies have to make up for the fact
that they were born less than good.

you remember the taste of sugared, cheap pleasure—
nutty buddies swiss-cake rolls oatmeal-cream pies
zebra cakes peanut butter crunch bars

bought later with change from your mother's purse—
fancy cakes devil squares banana twins

purchased in secret using the money a neighbor gave you—
the same one who watched you run through the sprinkler.

you consider this now over a piece of chocolate,
wondering again why some bodies were born good

and some bodies spend a lifetime making up for
the fact that they were born less than good.

the crime scene

was my body
I couldn't make sense
of the wounds
I saw—for years
no blood
or forensics to prove
their existence.
instead, I became
the witness,
unfolding
the yellow tape
wrapping it around
the words
caught in my throat
fantasies
confused by innocence
and pleasure
you see, I need
you to understand
I only wanted
people to love me.

the color wheel

as a child you learned the primary colors
red, yellow and blue

emotions too were simple
happy, sad or angry

secondary colors taught one lesson at a time
orange, green and purple

which was never enough for you—
who took in everything all at once, and yet,

somehow it was also too much, your sadness
occupied a vast spectrum of hues—

the regret of indigo blue,
the gray sky of silence

with clouds hovering over parched ground,
the imperceptible longing

hidden on a perfectly set table
covered by a chiffon, ivory runner

with long tendrils wrapped around your fingers
hiding the crimson sadness of shame

amidst the weighted evergreen passage of time.
you once tried to explain what you saw

and then learned that colors are only perceptions
which felt sad in a way you could not explain.

my maruska

I ask how we fit together—
our identical shapes of different sizes.

I remember watching as childhood
became the space between us

and then, breaking myself up into tiny parts,
I swallowed my aloneness

feeling it cover me like a mother's dress
three sizes too big, not understanding

I also carried the past inside of me,
filling up my field of vision, watching

as my life grew larger.

the void

emptiness grew between
what was given to you
and what was needed

in childhood, you remember
the feelings of
ineffable longing, air-filled

space, those unused
chambers of your heart
craving warm blood.

You trained your
touch-starved,
love-addicted self

to stay away from the edge
of what you wanted
but could not have.

Diagnoses

Decomposition

That night you woke to the scent of flesh, decomposing.
A light sulfur smell hung over your heavy body.
You shook your lover and asked if he could smell the same.
"The nights are short," he said, rolling over in bed.

In the morning, your fingers and toes were cold to the touch.
"Something inside of me is dying," I told him.
"You have everything you need," he said,
turning to the stove to fry eggs.

Driving, you notice the leaves are changing colors—
autumn's last stand is fiery and bright.

You wonder why some dying parts
evolved colorful displays, while others did not.

Is the breakdown of chlorophyll
self-cannibalism or self-preservation?

The geese fly south in a V formation.
You put your fingers out the car window and
contemplate air-filled space, the absence of matter,
the creation of vacuums and nothingness.

At work you observe small maggots
crawling out of your ears.
and gently pick the sticky nematodes off of your neck.
"I'm starting to decompose,"

you say out loud to no one in particular.
There was a time when life had intention and purpose.
Every day felt like a miracle.
Now you can hardly feel your own heart beating.

pudendum

pu·den·dum; /pyoō'dendəm/
the external genital organs
especially those of the female; vulva.

re-examining
the deepest examination, you learn
the medical term *pudenda*
means to be ashamed. you know
shame's first language
is spoken in the body.

simple words like yes and no
silent sounds, breath-holding—
expressions of suppressed emotion
felt by organs
fed by an internal plexus of nerves
confused by expectation and longing.

your heart
chased the leaves which fell
into the darkness
of *pudendum*.

Perspectives

Because you don't remember it that way
And you have a wife and daughters
Who you would never harm, or
A dear mother who recently passed

Away. Because lately I have noticed that
I work harder and you get paid
More. Because you are given special attention
for being a father, while mothers are watched

Carefully. Girls are told to be careful
Because you are like so many
Men. You see the affections won or lost
You don't see the desperate, trapped women

Escaping the right questions.
You proclaim, it is not personal
Because you don't know me
But you feel your wounds, your needs

Are personal. Because
You are the subject and I am the object
Because you have a narrative
And I am the narrator of this story.

crisis in the middle of life

in the morning you startle awake remembering that you forgot to schedule an orthodontic appointment for your child—pattern recognition in college taught you it was the tannins in the wine making you sick—putting blame on consumption during an evening of excess would have been too simple—you are not simple—now, if only the same purported wisdom could reveal the deeper purpose of your life and how to eschew this midlife unease—experts say that life satisfaction follows a u-shaped curve; happiness thrives in the young and the old with discontent in-between—you want to accept the fact that the simple and the mundane tasks now weave the tapestry of your life—nowadays, your mind buzzes with responsibility, imbibement refers to coffee and sleep deprivation causes you to dissociate—one glass of wine, maybe two on holidays—no indulgences, no indiscretions, fewer bad decisions and no headaches—your Facebook account reconnects you with an old friend who you suspect is buying Oxycontin illegally on the internet—contemplating your social media connections reminds you that the electric bill needs to be paid this month—you reflect on the fact that you will likely go to your grave not knowing the rush of heroin, then feel guilty for having had such a troubling thought—you try to be a good citizen and pay your late fines in advance when you return your overdue books this week at the library—sometimes, you consider all of the kinky things you wish you had been bold enough to try in your twenties before settling down and getting married—you think, part of your problem is that young people overestimate how happy they will be when they grow up—college should require a course on expectations and prepare you to lose all of your money, feel like a failure, have your heart broken, cry in front of your boss, back the car into a stationary object; and maybe, just maybe, one day you will find you are able to examine your life choices without a mid-life crisis—zoologists have shown that the Great Apes also get sad in middle age—you ponder this fact over one solitary glass of wine.

listen

"You never screamed for help?" —an attorney for
  D. J. Trump, questioning E. Jean Carroll in a rape case
against the 45th and 47th president

maybe I didn't always scream
when I wanted to be heard
you should know
that sometimes the tongue drowns
in the weighted language of silence
used to please others

maybe i didn't always scream
because I was dreaming
the mind heavy
with sleep paralysis—unmoving
the throat restrained with fear
not understanding
why the voice
was not attached to the body

lean in, listen
take out your ear plugs
and you will hear my voice
echo through the long chambers of time
I take in all that happens
I'm just not a screamer

smoke signals

maybe it wasn't a dream, or an illness
that brought visions of self-harm;

so often when they came you felt sick
torturing those dead parts,

with rope, guns, knives—how you ached
to see the blood run red rivers on your skin.

this is hard to write down,
nearly impossible to speak of—

to be seduced by the belief
that the creation of pain can settle pain;

to be tempted by the feeling
that self-harm settles memories of violence.

somehow, you always assumed
you were the problem—

now, you consider the possibility
that those visions were smoke signals

which came to warn you
that in your life, there was a problem.

the angle of my pelvis

lying on my back in that yoga position,
I imagine myself to be a dead, sexually vulnerable frog.
        "don't force your legs open," the teacher says,
as I ponder the evolutionary advantage of the female pelvis.
my viscera involuntarily contract and
I feel like a very small and a very cold amphibian
beached on the edge of a pond in mid-November.

pelvimetry measures the angles of the female pelvis.
theoretically, it can identify the body's adequacy for giving birth.
        "relax your legs open," the doctor says,
before jabbing something very cold and very metal
into the deepest cavity of my body
reasonably accessed without anesthesia.
(all in the name of good health and goodwill, of course)

as a young girl, I was amused
by the cross-legged attempts of sitting boys;
their knees flapping high in the air like butterfly wings.
at times, I had sympathy for their awkward bodies
lacking the natural flexibility of the female form.
sometimes, still, I am amused by men,
though the concern has gone.

evolutionary advantage is part truth and part perspective.
pelvimetry teaches that circumstances are also relevant.
"you should know better," women are often told,
as they then spend a lifetime trying to understand
how attention to the pelvis
can engender deep longing and excitement,
while also imprinting a lifetime of fear.

Onward to Camelot with *The Lady of Shalott*

—based on "The Lady of Shalott" by Alfred Lord Tennyson

Once I was charmed
by The Lady of Shalott,
lost as I was
on my way to Camelot.

Oh, The Lady of Shalott
in a remote castle tower
watched life as a reflection in the mirror
weaving for others, her joy just out of reach.

The promise of death for The Lady
if she left her dwelling or looked outside.
Living, it seemed, had cost
this woman her freedom.

From my own ivory tower I befriended The Lady
not a damsel in distress, still, from the window
I watched the wild birds flying circles
around the fortress I had built of other's expectations.

The Lady's hex, a whisper from an unknown source.
My own curse, subtle and given so long ago
I didn't recognize when it had arrived—
or perhaps, coming from voices so familiar, I came to trust it.

Then one day she wanted more,
"The mirror crack'd from side to side"
"The curse has come upon me," cried The Lady of Shalott
She then climbed in the boat that took her away.

And was found floating
down the river of Camelot. Dead.
On the boat engraved with her name—
"The Lady of Shalott."

How strange was the day I too wanted more.
Living life as a reflection had distorted my vision.
"Let me break my own mirror," I cried.
"I want to see the world with my own two eyes."

Banished from the tower, I climbed into the boat.
The river caressed my fingertips
as worn-out voices said,
"Don't rock the boat, don't take too much."

I saw her floating. Choose freedom, accept death.
I was floating. Choose death so the soul can live.
I am floating. Choose truth and a full life.
"God has enough victims," said the Lady of Shalott.

What I Understand of Helen and the Trojan War

In loud stillness
lives that strange desire
you have to screw all of your life up
to besiege faithfulness and virtue

knowing one day you might say to yourself,
"there was a time when I had everything,"
"until" or "and then,"
(and of course one always knows better)

but what you held onto
you also wanted to throw to the ground
anyways, with that angry habit you had
just to watch it crack, to deconstruct

to break itself up into hundreds of pieces
so all of Troy knew—your heart
as well as your resentful enslavement
to duty without desire

so too you yearned for right and wrong
as you bent over to pick up
unexploded bombs, shells and mines
those discarded weapons

which in your pocket were simply too heavy
for you to carry.

The Peach Stand

In the brightness of day, sunlight burns the eyes
and you buy peaches from a roadside stand.

In your car, you inhale the sweetness
savoring one and then another, as if tasting for the first time.

Their ripeness reminds you of pleasure
and the blossoms that birthed pleasure, once.

In the rearview mirror you see salty, wet fruit juice
watering your cheeks;
imagining
the dusty hands of farm workers,
the fragility of peach skins and marriage,
the inevitability of change.

You recall with hope the buds that bloomed in spring
trying to understand the ache which has

taken up residence in your heart; remembering
the kiss last night that took three attempts to complete;
wondering

about lovers who cannot find each other in the dark.
After a pause, you move the peaches to the trunk and
drive yourself home.

nourishment

you are watched so closely
the full vision of you is not seen
as another person praises you
for losing weight.

in this form,
you find yourself shrinking.
becoming the shadows
of what others see.

"tell me how," they say
"I want that," they say
"you must be so happy,
  they say "to see this result."

your mind ponders this diet
of unreasonable expectations,
mealtimes filled with work
and tables empty of nourishment.

your body watches emotion
take residence in your gut
knowing there are many twists, turns
and places to hide.

it is always the eyes which bend light
and bring the world into focus.
"look here," you want to say,
"if you have questions for me."

The Dead Bird

That morning I saw a dead bird.
I imagined what she saw
or didn't see
as she flew towards herself
hitting the glass with a thud—
a detritus of soft flesh and light feathers
splayed on the ground beneath the window.
Confetti, the afterparty, she won't remember;
the price of her own self-examination
beckoning to her, that morning
mistaking her own reflection
for some other, enemy bird.
In the end, she did not think.

Take care

Because your mind wasn't always the best caretaker for this body.

Because your body was ill-fitting, you sometimes wanted to take it off and give it away.

Because your head wasn't screwed on right, you couldn't stop facing your flaws.

Because your head always wanted to be right, you never wanted to face your flaws.

Because you found it so hard to look at yourself in the mirror with your eyes wide open.

Because of your tendency to shape-shift, you thought you could become what others wanted.

Because of that lump in your throat, you found it hard to speak in a way that made you feel heard.

Because the medical term for "a lump in the throat" is *globus pharyngeus.*

Because doctors usually don't know the cause or how to help someone with *globus pharyngeus.*

Because you were keeping your chin up, you found there was something you wanted to get off of your chest.

Because your heart went out with the tide and didn't come back.

Because it is heart wrenching to find your heart's not in the right place—especially if you know you put it there, once.

Because one day you found out that all meat-eating animals have a gallbladder.

Because those butterflies in your stomach give you a gut punch, a gut feeling that things could be different.

Because your constitution is a jigsaw puzzle with bent and missing pieces.

Because your eyes are sore from trying to see a new vision.

Because the human eye can focus on fifty different objects every second.

Because all of the sacred texts say the same thing.

Because you are ready for a new way of being in this world.

Because when you take a deep breath and your feet touch the floor, you are reminded that sometimes the body is the caretaker for the mind.

Because your body exists as a part of this world, not separate from it.

The Universe

In the emptiness of space
all around
I saw an open field
of abandoned touch.

I watched the departure
of neutrinos and cosmic rays
making myself small to fit the interior
of forgotten places;
those deep holes of blackness,
with electromagnetic solitary fields.

In my darkness,
I inhabited the space
which had long been emptied
of all the night stars.

The Lesson

confused
by perception,
the girl became
her dark thoughts,

in the same way
the earnest
are so easily deceived
by their best teachers.

ad sanadum

In the stories

buried under you and over time,

are the words with instructions on
how pain can break a person
with shards of glass, with whispers

you were taught how to hide
how to become small, except
you could not disappear in that body,
you could not unlive the feelings
that came with being alive.

Today, your blistered hands burn
as you hold onto this earth
tethered by your grief;

like a kite tied to a signpost
with each gust of wind,
the love and loss

steal the ground out from under you,
they take your breath away.

Fulfurite

Women have curves, you said
unseeing

the well-defined angle of my clavicle,
the flat bridge of my nose,
the sharpness of my tongue,
and the clarity of my vision.

Women are soft, you said
unknowing

the toughness of my skin which can scatter the sting of pain
just as lightning strikes the ground of a high desert landscape,
fusing sand grains into otherworldly glass sculptures
diffusing the power of a charge.

Of this strength
even Charles Darwin spoke.

dolls

in childhood
you assigned humanistic qualities
to inanimate objects

unprepared for the knowledge
that your toys were not real
you then spent years

in the stillness of painted faces
absorbing the static creation of identity,
even learning how to make love
from the outside of your body.

in adulthood
the reckoning finally came
when you admitted

that your dolls were never real
but in your body
you are.

*** It's hard to be real.

The Feel of Rain

I used to dream I was so strong,
Nothing could harm me.
I hardened under loss and told myself
To stop wanting touch.

I used to pride myself on my ability to be alone,
To withstand the incessant ache of loneliness
Frozen between my shoulder blades.
I never needed anyone to help me.

I used to practice the art of disappearing,
The exercise of becoming what was needed.
I kept a careful eye on my reflection
And changed myself to fill my image.

I used to hone the skill of denying discomfort,
Rejecting the feeling that I was dying on the inside.
Walking in a cold rain I turned towards the sky
And told myself I didn't feel the water.

These days my body no longer
Wants to protect my mind from its stories.
When rain runs off my face
I see the rivulets of water as my very own tears.

The Feel of Light

when i was young
i sat in a dark closet praying
i could learn
how to make my other people happy.

today I sat in the wet grass
absorbing sunlight, praying
I will learn
how to let myself be happy.

Dear Teenager,

To the girl who is always wanting, yearning, I wish you knew more about this thing called enough—To the girl who steps into perfectionism like a dress two sizes too small, who plans her life so she can give it away, who thinks there is valor in sacrificing the biggest parts of herself . . . if I could go back, I would tell you about park benches—I would tell you that it's okay to sit down once in a while even if you were not planning on it—even if others tell you to keep on going—I would tell you that the day might come when you choose to give up a job in an office with big windows just so you stand a chance of taking a break once in a while—I would share with you how good it feels to eat your lunch and then tell you how much your body craves being outside—I would tell you that one day while taking a walk on your lunch break, you might even surprise yourself by sitting down on a park bench—I would tell you about the sadness that comes when a person suddenly notices that all of the autumn leaves have already fallen from the trees—I would tell you that even with the sadness, bittersweet is the best flavor—I would explain that enoughness is like the wind, it can't be observed directly though sometimes you can feel it brushing up against your skin, whispering in your ear, pushing through the emptiness—I would tell you that life is hard and the phrase, "it could be worse," is not the same as "good enough"—I would tell you that one day we both might find ourselves sitting on a park bench with our hands in our pockets holding onto the softness of an imperfect body—surprised, somehow, that all of this felt like enough.

obscure

I am lost. I look behind me
in an effort to understand

how my thoughts have led me to here.
I try but find I cannot fill in that empty space.

In the light of day, I am not seen.
This tells me I must be what is missing

The brain has a map.
My brain longs for what is absent.

I know the human body is opaque
so, I cradle my shadow.

Experts say that even in the dark
the brain observes its own body moving.

I feel the weight of my darkness.
I cannot move.

Light reflects off of surfaces and enters the eyes.
I see because of the light.

Most days I find that I am still lost.

the size of wanting

that phrase—I want
felt too big.
"so," I said, "whatever"
or, "whatever you prefer"
not understanding
that offering without wanting
can leave a person hungry—
starving.

despite everything I took in
I could not fill up
my longing
so I became small
to shrink my wanting,
to fit my understanding.
I cut myself into pieces
and then I swallowed them whole.

something to get off your chest

there you go again
feeling your chest
cave in on itself
you can't help but think
maybe it's your breasts
everyone has a name for
those white fleshy mounds
which have been
weighing you down
your whole life
pulling your shoulders forward—
"look here," you want to say
gesturing towards
your hazel-flecked eyes
even as your "jugs, knockers and ta-tas"
cast spells on lovers and babies
capturing the gaze of strangers
(perhaps you did or did not want this to happen)
you remember when
your 8th-grade math teacher
would look at your "boobs"
(that's what the 7th-grade boys called them)
and not at your face
as you answered questions in algebra class
in college, your friends
affectionately nicknamed them "the girls"
sometimes you wished
you were flat like a runway model
then there would be nothing to hold onto
nothing to let go of
"look at the way clothing sways on her body,"
people would say.

distance

from the viewfinder
on the edge of the cliff
I saw: a sandhill crane,
people gathered together in crowds,
but not the field of loneliness
which was all around me.

through the lens of distance,
I viewed continuous stars
stretched across the night sky
with the knowledge
that their nearest neighbors
are actually light years away.

the inception

tell me about the beginning—
the feeling one has

when they were left behind
under a frozen layer of snow.

tell me how one grows
in near total darkness.

imagine I was there with you,
dreaming of a seed's first opening

watching my own heartbeat
slow and then stop.

the stillness of winter
brought me to you;

digging for roots,
begging for nourishment,

seeking forgiveness,
asking for everything.

On impermanence

you are not tied down.
Adrift, you imagine
all the different ways
parachutes fail
under the weight of
aloneness,
you observe
that falling bodies
are so rarely saved
by all the world's gifts.
With no other choice,
you put your hand out
on the way down
hoping to find a way
to soften the landing.

maybe

we could leave things right where they are
and call this good enough
because nothing is changing anytime soon
this I know, *for sure.*

maybe I'm just one of those people
who deals in the "good enough"
even if it means I'm carrying a mineshaft of loneliness
from my heart to my toes.

sometimes, I think, "it could be worse"
and maybe that's the same as "good enough."

you see, I am willing to overlook all those times
I went to bed hungry, starving,
wanting for something I couldn't quite name
waking up to find I was chewing on the tips of my fingers
sucking so hard on the inside of my forearm
I left red marks on my skin, just as in childhood
when I knew nothing about hickies and lovemaking
and the hurt that comes from love—

except, even then I knew that pain can feel good
if you let it,
if you are not afraid of it,
if you touch it,
if you sink into it and swaddle it up like a newborn baby.

so, maybe dealing in the "good enough"
is the same as holding on real tight to sadness
wrapping her up in a stretchy blanket
saying, "I've got you babe, don't worry."
I'll take care of you.
I won't get rid of you,
because this is my life
and that's good enough.

unraveling

one day you learn

that the becoming
          is the undoing

not the creation of
          who you thought you were

while trying to please others
          you lost sight of

your true reflection
          as it shined in the mirror

of your heart.

Seasonal Depression

What would you think
if I told you
that I don't like sunshine?

The beating drum of it,
the way sweat rains
down and dilutes the world

exposing the soft vulnerability
of all our shadows
with its bright arrogance—

daylight becomes
yet another expectation
forcing a downwards gaze.

You must know,
my thoughts
flourish in the dark.

tailspin

one day
you find yourself
on the edge of a cliff,
a precipice,
weeping with the stories
moving within
and all around you.
falling,
you admit that
you were never
aerodynamic or graceful,
only human.
you ask for help
and voices echo
within the container
of your imagination.
you contemplate
the stages of flight,
make deals with God,
succumb to psychotherapy
and medications
and time.
falling,
your heart sinks
and your arms reach out for comfort—
which has always been
just beyond your reach—
along with parachutes,
feathers and unconditional love.
the colors blur together
and you are confused by the person
you are meant to be.
except, you know
that you are here now,
still falling.

Storytelling

There I was
writing out my story.

And again,
I thought

what the hell,
it still hurts.

After all this time,
why would

it still hurt?
And then

I thought
well, at least

I am here
writing out my story.

You know
there was a time

it hurt too much
to do that.

The Effects of Climate Change

The national weather service issues an excessive heat warning:

Hot, humid temperatures are uncomfortable
and some people will be harmed
if precautions are not taken.

People will want things from me today,
things which I cannot give:
Hands which can stop the clocks of time,
Answers to questions which begin with the word why—

For this, I will apologize for seeing the chasm
between what is desired and what is truly possible.

Instead,

I ask the world to teach me about unconditional love—
to speak without words, to touch without fingertips.

I ask to see and be seen over and over again—
even in the midst of suffering,
even with the harsh glare of it,
even after others have looked away.

Admittedly, I contribute to climate change
But I do not control the weather.

Spring Wind

It was strange to see my soul
opening its arms to the same body
it had rejected in childhood,

just as my body opened the door
      so that my soul could feel
            the freedom of a warm spring wind.

I saw something special that year
in the timid beauty of the crocuses
as they broke through the dirt seeking sun,

the same bulbs I had forgotten about
before the cold of winter made it impossible
            for all living things to grow.

what security feels like

because I wanted to feel safe
I built myself a house—
a home with four walls,
two windows, a roof and a door.

because I wanted to feel safe
I covered the glass windows with plywood
and reinforced the walls
with sandbags and layers of brick.

at night, I barricaded the door with furniture
and I turned off the lights
so it looked like I was not home.
all of this, because I wanted to feel safe.

despite these protections,
I could still sense the danger out there—
and one day my heart would not quiet
because it wanted to feel safe.

so I became small again
and held on so I could not come undone.
I pushed my fingernails into the foundation
under the floor in that house and I started digging.

Seeds

Seven date palm trees (Phoenix dactylifera) have been grown
from 2000-year-old seeds that were found in the Judean desert
near Jerusalem. The seeds—the oldest ever germinated—were
discovered in caves in an ancient palace built by King Herod in the
first century BCE.

Crossing terrain of the familiar
within myself, worn out voices

whispered, "you, you
will always be unworthy,

of this, you will never be free."
To go further, to survive

I dragged my bound soul
across years with rivers of yearning

to find the cave holding
the shadows of my existence—

those discarded remains
not fit for the light of living:

broken shells, decaying bones,
of emptiness and being emptied,

legacies of silence, my solitude,
I opened you up to me. And there,

in the radiance of darkness
were the seeds for a deserving life.

on longing

"Our hearts are restless until they rest in you."
—St. Augustine (397–400 CE)

fernweh is the German word
for farsickness. a distant pain,
that traveler's ache,
a desire for unseen places.

some people dream
of lush green forests, ancestral
grounds, fantastical landscapes
like Tolkien's middle earth.

you know insatiable feelings—
the scent of a flower you have not found,
the sight of a songbird you have heard,
but never seen,
from behind the open window.

the more of life you take in
the greater this hunger becomes.

some days, you fear drowning
in the beauty of a full night sky.
other days, the absence of emptiness
haunts the chambers of your heart
teaching you about the pain of unconditional love.

you hear an infant cry out in the night—
the end is the beginning—
and you wake to find the hand on your face
belongs to your very own body.

fernweh
is the opposite of homesickness.
you are a traveler who does not know home,
you breathe into the empty bags you carry.

tug of war

I wish we could talk
about that feeling
of wanting to stay
and wanting to go
at the same time;
the way the mind
plays with abandonment
drawing attention
to the emptiness,
the open space
surrounded by
the perimeter of your life;
facing the feeling that
whatever you take in
it will never be enough—
just like the satin-lined edge
of the cotton blanket
you once held onto
rubbing the softest part
between your fingers
you wanted the entirety
to be like that.
I wish we could talk
about how one grieves
for something
they never actually had;
the longing that
morphs into fast breathing
the anxiety that seeps
from your wounds
unraveling to destroy
the very thing
you hold onto.

I wish we could talk about
how difficult it is
to be present for life
even as death pulls on you
day after day.

on letting go of fear of drowning

it was the strangest thing
to acknowledge
that you no longer
feared drowning, because
you recalled that your body
already knew how to swim.

furthermore,
the people, the responsibilities
you thought were giving you buoyancy—
all this time,
had only been
weighing you down.

once you were no longer
afraid of the creatures
living in the cold dark waters
below the surface
you were finally able to let go
and enjoy the freedom that comes

from swimming in the ocean.

adaptation

let's go back to the beginning
if you can imagine
roaming buffalo, wild horses
huddled together before the storm.

let's go back to a time
when this was enough,
when our DNA could absorb
the direct pounding of the wind and rain.

let's go back to a time
when storms did not summon
an impending sense of doom.

I was raised behind 12-inch walls
with double-paned windows.

I was assured my life was safe
not understanding why
I felt afraid so much of the time,

or why I felt alone
even when I was standing in the herd;
unable to understand
why I needed sleeping pills to sleep

or why I didn't sleep.
let's go back to a time
when we let ourselves feel all of the
storm
because it was in our DNA to do so.

the practice of wanting a life

I always thought those two words—*I want*—
were a prelude to something childishly selfish, as in,
I want more ice cream; I want to stay up late tonight.

And then, I felt every square inch of my adult body
vibrate with the loneliness that once silenced
that lovely childlike sense of wanting.

And then, the permission to say those two words,
I want, became a transition point—
a passageway to reclaim my very own life.

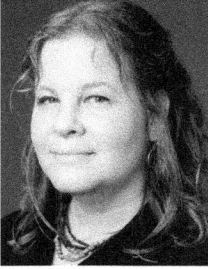

JACQUELINE S. REDMER M.D. practices family medicine and palliative care in the Driftless Region of southwest Wisconsin. She is also the mother of three school-aged girls. She started writing poetry during the Covid pandemic to steady herself during the brief pauses of a busy life. Her writing has been published in *Examined Life Journal*, *The Intima Journal*, *Bramble*, *Wisconsin Poets Calendar*, and *Kevin MD Blog*. She recently completed the Columbia University Narrative Medicine CPA program and has pursued creative writing courses through Stanford University Continuing Studies Program. Her favorite place to write is in the backyard sauna.

Shanti Arts

Nature · Art · Spirit

Please visit us online
to browse our entire book catalog,
including poetry collections and fiction,
books on travel, nature, healing, art,
photography, and more.

Also take a look at our highly regarded art
and literary journal, *Still Point Arts Quarterly*,
which may be downloaded for free.

www.shantiarts.com

www.ingramcontent.com/pod-product-compliance
Lightning Source LLC
Chambersburg PA
CBHW070008100426
42741CB00012B/3153